The Holistic

Depress:

Healthy Habits and Holistic Remedies to Stop Depression

Book Five of the Healthiest Life Possible Series

The "Fire Lotus" Seal of Quality

DevelopedLife.com prides itself on high-quality content. We are against the trend on Amazon / Kindle of cheap, outsourced content written by non-authors.

Free Supplemental Booklet: Right now you can check out www.developedlife.com/subscribe and receive a free copy of the booklet "**10 Success Techniques to Master Your Life**" for those who desire to create optimal life philosophies. This is an important resource to have alongside this book.

You can also visit the exclusive mailing list for natural health and wellness by going to www.developedlife.com/andreasilver, where you can stay in contact with Andrea personally, and get another cool free book: "**The 20 Most Deceptive Health Foods**".

Table of Contents

Introduction

Depression, typically characterized into minor and major depressive disorders, is a chronic mood imbalance that may be related to both psychological and chemical factors. Depression can be a severe illness that interferes with quality of life and damages the ability to even get through the day.

There are many things people don't understand about depression, and while the chemical factors can be regulated with medication, the origins of depression exist on a case-by-case basis; with factors that range from genetics to psychological trauma.

One factor that is even less understood by mainstream medicine is geography. Depression rates greatly differ based on where a person lives. Certain countries are rife with high depression, while other countries are categorized as very low on the "happiness index", with depression one of the signs of an unhappy people.

For me personally, I don't think its rocket-science to figure out why some places are just plain happier. Recently, I was touring the beautiful city of Prague. I was amazed how much higher quality the food was compared to the United States. Even at the little gas station markets—there was cheap whole wheat bread, fresh fruits and vegetables, and very few processed foods.

In addition, there was something very lively about the atmosphere. The architecture was amazing and immediately elevated my spirits just by stepping out the door. There was a lot more activity on the streets than in places like Phoenix, Arizona--and there was a general free-spirited atmosphere.

I hypothesized that people from such a beautiful environment have to, in general, be happier about life compared to back at home. In addition, such an abundance of fresh, organic food could have some effect, as well. So I did some research. Per capita depression rates in Czech Republic are around 8% of the population[1], compared to U.S.

depression levels that hover around 18% (or more than twice the amount). The United States, it turns out, is one of the most depressed countries on Earth!

Of course, I don't think this is simply a matter of really nice countries like the Czech Republic being happier. Many other places far less beautiful than Prague are also less depressed than the United States, too. Almost anywhere you go in Europe is significantly less depressed, with depression rates lingering between 6 and 9%. And, this problem is also far less severe in most Southeast Asian countries, as well.

So am I saying more than half of the depression of America is caused by a poor culture? Well, I think this is very possible. In the USA, I believe we take natural depression cures for granted, we rely too much on chemical models of the human mind, and we don't take a hard look at our lifestyles as the thing that's making us so afflicted.

Today we live in a culture where it's "a pill for every ill", and depression pills are among the most popular. 1 in 10 Americans over age 12 are currently prescribed antidepressants, according to the CDC[2]. Among various other factors, this may blind people to making the needed lifestyle changes to precipitate greater happiness.

And, anybody with any experience in the medical profession can tell you that pharmaceutical salespeople aggressively market their products to doctors, creating an environment where it's in a doctor's best interest to suggest pharmaceutical alternatives to common sense, natural or holistic remedies.

To illustrate this point further, a European friend of mine applied for a work program in Canada (she is from Norway). In order to be accepted for the job, she had to undergo a psychiatric evaluation to make sure she was "fit to live in the country" (maybe they believed Norwegian's lack of sunshine predisposes them to mental ills and sluggishness).

---

[1] http://ec.europa.eu/health/ph_determinants/life_style/mental/docs/Czech.pdf
[2] http://www.cdc.gov/nchs/data/databriefs/db76.htm

"Is there anything bothering you in your life?"
"Not really, I'm quite happy," she replied.
"Nothing at all? Do you miss home?"
"Well, yes, sometimes I do miss home quite a bit."
"So you're sad?"
'Sometimes, I suppose."
"I see. I am going to prescribe you this antidepressant called…"

She, of course, got a good laugh out of it. She never fulfilled her prescription, and explained how she realized then that "it was true" what they said about the West—pharms are passed out like M&Ms. This is of particular concern considering the number of side-effects that these drugs create, including even the potential for *increased* depression and suicidal tendencies.

We'll return to the issues of culture and geography later. In the meantime, we are going to explore many other sources and (potential) natural and holistic depression cures that you can apply as a solid strategy to get better.

For the purposes of this book, I'm not advocating to get off your meds or to not take them. There are many shades of truth in the mainstream medical world that we can't ignore in order to become alternative health extremists. All I am suggesting, however, are two things:

- The first is that anti-depressant drugs were intended by the scientists who made them to work as a treatment to stabilize mood while undergoing psychiatric care. This means weaning off them eventually, instead of hooking patients for life.

- The second is that there are literally dozens of things a person can do *before* beginning anti-depressant treatment, to see if those things fix the problem before beginning chemical solutions.

I am not a doctor, all I can do is provide to you suggestions that you can accept or toss in the junk pile. However, I will say one thing: I am sorely disappointed by many Western doctors who do not do anything more than cough up expensive prescriptions. They rarely suggest dietary or lifestyle changes, and many live by the mantra that "diet, nutrition and regular therapies do not work as anything other than a preemptive strategy. When the disease is happening, there is no cure but treatment and pills". This is one line of thinking in the medical field, that despite being recognized by every medical school graduate, I happen to know is just plain wrong and basically delusional.

Eastern medicine, which is to say hospitals in areas from Cambodia to China to Central Asia and even Central Europe are far more attuned to the body, the mind, and the environment. Why Western doctors are so far behind them is truly sad, indeed!

Without further ado, let's get started:

Chapter One – Do You Have Depression?

A common myth about depression is that it's one of those illnesses that you're acutely aware of once you have it. While it's true that many people recognize it immediately, and may say something to the effect of "I feel depressed this day / week / month," there are other times that depression may manifest without the victim understanding that it's the source of problems.

Examples of hidden depressive symptoms include:

- Sudden loss of interest in your job, hobbies, or friends.
- Changes in sleep patterns.
- Sudden irritability
- Anger and hostility
- Onset of reckless behavior
- Low energy levels
- Feelings of worthlessness or negative self-imagery.

But everyone experiences some of these emotions, right?

The answer is yes—everyone does, presuming you are a human and not a Star Trek cyborg. The odds are, you're experiencing what doctors call **minor depressive disorder**. This could occur spontaneously, but most psychiatrists would link it to a specific occurrence. As an example, a sudden change can precipitate it, like moving to a new city. Or, it could be the remnants of grief that may have occurred from loss (like death) that occurred even a long time ago.

Most of the time, minor depression goes away. Usually, some type of change is needed to rectify the situation. This is usually about the time that someone may start thinking about when to punch in their two week vacation time.

However, sometimes minor depression graduates into something worse.

Major and Moderate Depression

Two weeks or more of sustained depression may warrant a doctor to diagnose a patient with major depression[3]. Various therapies are usually recommended, including an anti-depressant prescription.

There are some distinctions between moderate and major (severe) depression. Moderate depression can include sustained feelings of anger, agitation, despair, grief, or worthlessness that begin to interfere with daily activities. Major and severe depression takes this a step further and could include dangerous behaviors, leading a doctor to be concerned about things like the threat of suicide.

An example of major depression could be when a person is paralyzed by their mental state, unable to leave their house or otherwise experiencing a level of catharsis that becomes self-destructive by nature. Sometimes if it is not the sufferer him or herself who will go to a doctor, it will be a friend or family member who will try to seek help; sometimes as a matter of emergency.

Chronic Depression (Dysthermia)

Another classification of depression ranges more on the mild level, but is marked by persistence. Dysthermia is when those milder but noticeable depressive symptoms and negative feelings never really go away; but a person carries them constantly. According to the National Institutes of Health, 1.5% of Americans suffer from dysthermia. However, my personal opinion is that this number is probably much higher than that.

---

[3] http://www.webmd.com/depression/guide/depression-types

Bipolar Depression

As with major depression, this can be a serious diagnosis, and strong mood stabilizers (usually of the lithium variety) may be prescribed for patients who are affected by a bipolar disorder. Probably more than other diagnoses, bipolar depression (once known as manic depression) can be identified more clearly as a chemical disruption in the brain. Sufferers swing wildly from high to low, with the lowest points resembling major / severe depression, which can pose a serious risk to the person. Bipolar disorder may require extensive medical help if you are diagnosed as such.

Seasonal Affective Disorder

Wintery climates without much sun appear to precipitate higher cases of depression, and certainly some people are more vulnerable than others. Sunlight helps the body to release serotonin, a neurotransmitter that scientists believe is important for mood regulation. Aside from issues related to wintery months, it would seem obvious that a serotonin deficiency could arise from excessive time indoors (such as at an office) without spending adequate time outside.

Postpartum Depression

Mothers who have recently conceived a child are well-known to experience signs of depression, which can sometimes be so severe that it leads to self-harm. Doctors believe PTD is related to hormonal changes in the body after finishing pregnancy. This is another example of a very biologically driven depression, although the symptoms could also be exacerbated by the stress involved with having a new child.

Psychotic Depression

Another serious form. Depression may accompany a major mental illness, like psychosis. Hallucinations, fits of rage and chronic paranoia could also be merged with major depressive symptoms, rendering a person a danger to him or herself or others. I think it's fairly obvious if a loved one is suffering from an example this extreme; and they will require immediate mental care.

Habits That Follow Depression

One of the dangers of untreated depression is the adoption of harmful habits as a way for the sufferer to cope. This may include alcoholism, drugs, or even food addiction. It's not uncommon for people who suffer from some form of substance addiction to also be suffering from depression. Typically the substance abuse is a symptom of the depression; and recovery depends on treating the depression first, as even if the addiction wanes, it may manifest in another way if that person continues to be mentally ill.

Reimagining Depression Holistically

The types of depression I've listed so far, as you can see, vary significantly in scope and range, and there are certainly some classifications that seem to be more physiological versus psychological. Most commonly, the types of depression that occurs are minor, moderate and severe depressive disorders. But how do we understand exactly what depression even is? In academia, I've found there is a back-and-forth between people who claim everything is related to pharmacological explanations and cures, and others who say it's purely psychiatric—it's all in the mind.

I think the best way to think of depression is to look into the root of the word itself. *De-pression*, which means something that is *compacted* or *compressed* together. In this case, a sense of pressure has been put under your happiness or sense of well-being.

Therefore, to cure *de-pression* you must, in a sense, *recompress*, which is defined as a renewal of the regular atmosphere. Depression, as it's originally defined, is thus a very temporary, atmospheric, circumstantial event. As with many things in Western culture, this condition is seen as something that's "bad" and should be immediately eliminated—but is this true? We could also look at depression holistically, and discover that the symptoms may not actually be as negative as we think.

If something in your environment or lifestyle is creating a *depression* against your well-being, the symptoms we attribute to depression is a mental and physiological response to it. It could even be considered your subconscious mind crying out for help. So the question is, should we suppress that feeling or listen to it, and think of a way to make the specific change that our mind and body requires?

For this reason, there really should be two types of "cures" to think about: the first are ways to alleviate the symptoms in relation to diet, nutrients, and chemicals, and the second is to figure out what parts of your life need to be fixed to restore mental equilibrium. Despite what Western medicine would have you believe, we are not robots and our consciousness is a real thing, and we must pay attention to our environment and personal desires and needs, because sometimes the primary culprit behind depression is merely a life that is out of sync with the way it's supposed to be.

An example could be a bad job, a bad relationship, a lack of friends and social contact, or just a situation that feels hopeless, where you are not living up to the potential you deserve. Even if you are not consciously recognizing these problems, they may still exist, and your physiology and emotions may start to alert you that something's wrong even before you are fully aware of what the problem is.

As I talked about before, maybe the reason that depression rates are higher in some countries is because those cultures have populations that are less in sync. I sometimes feel in American cities that our ambition and drive toward success could have a drawback when we neglect social, holistic and spiritual components of our lives. We seem to pride ourselves on the "Every man / woman for him/herself" concept, but this flows against our innate desire for family and companionship. I can't help but wonder if just the very environment of a high competition enterprise doesn't create subconscious wounds on most people.

If you think you have depression, consider before you lament too much that the depression is really a warning sign that something needs to change. Even if you took the necessary steps to stifle the depression, without the environmental factors taken into consideration, then you're really just treating it in a palliative way by not thinking about the source of the depression. Hopefully as this book continues, you'll figure out some strategies to focus on the source and not the symptoms.

Hey! You reading this! Did you receive your <u>free</u> gift yet?

I don't want you to get fooled anymore at the checkout aisle. That's why I've created a free e-book to reveal deceptive health foods that consumers need to beware of.

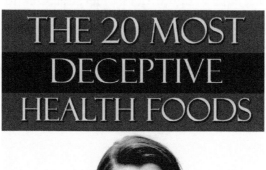
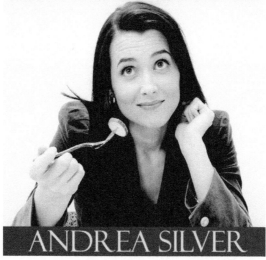

I'm giving it away right now for readers. You can get it at www.developedlife.com/andreasilver.

Chapter Two – Dietary Depression Cures

A 2008 report by the Indian Journal of Psychiatry has made it clear that nutrition and depression are actually closely linked together, and it's becoming an increasingly important topic even in mainstream psychiatry. Here is one excerpt:

"When we take a close look at the diet of depressed people, an interesting observation is that their nutrition is far from adequate. They make poor food choices and selecting foods that might actually contribute to depression. Recent evidence suggests a link between low levels of serotonin and suicide. It is implicated that lower levels of this neurotransmitter can, in part, lead to an overall insensitivity to future consequences, triggering risky, impulsive and aggressive behaviors which may culminate in suicide, the ultimate act of inwardly directed impulsive aggression." (Indian J Psychiatry. 2008 Apr-Jun; 50(2): 77–82.)[4].

Your diet could be either a partial factor that exacerbates existing depression symptoms, or it could be a prime culprit. Either way, your diet's effect on your emotional / mental health is something that nutritionists have always known—and have tried to warn people about. One of the very first steps to curing depression is to consider what you're eating, so let's delve into the basics:

Tryptophan and Amino Acids

Firstly, there is increasing research that suggests what you eat can have an effect on your mood. Earlier we mentioned the neurotransmitter serotonin that can be activated by sunlight. Another trigger of serotonin is tryptophan, which we more famously are aware of as the property that allegedly creates drowsiness consuming

---

[4] http://www.ncbi.nlm.nih.gov/pmc/articles/PMC2738337/

turkey (this is actually a myth, as turkey contains no more tryptophan than chicken).

However, while meats (poultry, or any protein dish) and certain plants (like seaweed, turnips and pumpkin) contain tryptophan, amino acids are required to carry it to the brain in-order to produce the active chemical we want, known as 5-HTP. So in addition to increasing tryptophan in our diets, what we really need are foods rich in amino acids to activate it. Therefore, this is just one reason to consider a diet rich in whole foods, fruits, and vegetables. In addition, carbohydrates also provide the energy needed to maintain these cellular processes, and some studies have linked low carbohydrate diets to lower tryptophan and decreased mood. So, consider increasing your intake of "good" carbs—whole wheat bread, seed, nuts and beans—in addition to foods with tryptophan.

Omega Fatty Acids

One of the more exciting developments in natural depression remedies comes from omega 3 fatty acids. Found plentifully in oily fish like sardines, dairy (eggs), seeds, and nuts—omega fatty acids are quickly becoming a staple food among health experts, not only for cardiovascular health, anti-aging properties, but also apparently brain health.

A 2006 Norwegian study brought together 22,000 participants to study the effects of omega-3 supplement cod liver oil. Among their findings, they discovered that cod liver users were 30% less likely to develop depression[5].

A second study done by the Royal College of Surgeons in Ireland further supported this finding[6]. 49 patients with a history of chronic depression and a tendency for self-harm were gathered and tested

[5] Raeder MB, Steen VM, Vollset SE, Bjelland I. Associations between cod liver oil use and symptoms of depression: The Hordaland Health Study. J Affect Disord. 2006 Dec 18.
[6] Hallahan B, Hibbeln JR, Davis JM, Garland MR. Omega-3 fatty acid supplementation in patients with recurrent self-harm. Single-centre double-blind randomised controlled trial. Br J Psychiatry. 2007 Feb;190:118-22.

with omega-3 supplementation, while providing a control group with a placebo. At the end of the 12-week course, the group that received the true supplementation showed "significant" improvement, with decreased depression, stress, and suicidal tendencies.

Hypotheses why omega acids help center around the fact the human brain is an extremely fatty organ (60% fat, and also very high cholesterol, so be careful if for some strange reason you enjoy eating brains). The structure of the brain thus depends on nutritious fats entering the body, as this is what brain cells need to communicate. If there is a lack of proper fats in a diet, then various cognitive functions could be threatened, including proper hormonal regulation. Feelings like hyperactivity and mood swings could result in a depression diagnosis, and it could be caused by an unhealthy brain.

This concept could apply on a larger scale to your, too. As "we are what we eat", a diet that neglects brain health could inevitably cause emotional difficulties. My suggestion? Start cutting out bad, saturated fats and greatly increase your omega-3 levels. Aside from nuts and eggs, another excellent source is avocado; which contains many other health benefits, as well. As a first step to tackling your depression from a dietary point of view, something as simple as daily servings of a nutritious food can be surprisingly effective. 1-2 mashed avocados with lemon juice makes a great lunch.

Selenium

An overlooked mineral in our diets is selenium, which is typically found in soil and spring water. Our bodies require a small amount of it, 55 micrograms per day, to help with important metabolic processes. Typically we fulfill this requirement in our day to day foods, but it is possible to become selenium deficient.

The reason selenium is considered a possible depression aid is because of a Texas Tech University study that increased selenium amounts to 200 micrograms per day among depressed elderly patients with satisfactory results, and there are also studies that appear to link low selenium with mood disorders.

It is not recommended to take selenium supplements, as selenium toxicity has been reported. However, as is usually the case, fresh foods allow easier absorption of minerals, and your daily intake can increase just by changing your diet a little bit.

The following foods not only increase selenium, but should provide some omega-3 fatty acids as well, so you're killing two birds with one stone:

- Brazil nuts
- Cashews
- Almonds
- Various beans and legumes
- And seafood (try oysters for an additionally healthy dose of zinc)

Turmeric

Studies have shown that turmeric, a primary ingredient in Indian curry and many other exotic meals, is also a potent "brain food" that helps with gene activation in the brain. This means stronger neurotransmitter signals / neuron function, including increased cellular battery power (mitochondria). Stronger brain signals, of course, means a stronger signal for our consciousness to use the brain properly, which means better balanced emotions. One recipe for a daily dose of turmeric is to add a couple of teaspoons to a glass of organic milk; creating "golden milk" which is a famous natural health remedy.

Making a B Vitamin Rich Diet

One of the best dietary techniques to immediately combat depression, according to numerous doctors and nutritionists, is one high in vitamin B-12, B-6, and folate. According to Harvard University, a B vitamin deficiency can be "sneaky and harmful", leading to behavioral changes that include paranoia, hallucinations, a difficult time processing thoughts, and depression[7]. So, could B vitamins be a culprit for what's making you depressed? Most people get adequate B vitamin levels from their diets; however, if your diet is not properly managed, it's possible you could be limiting your intake. Here are some risk factors:

- Are you a vegan? If so, you need to be eating enough foods fortified with B12, namely fortified breads and grains. Unfortunately, most B12 sources include dairy and meat, and without taking care to eat fortified foods, it's easy for a vegan to become deficient.

- Do you have any issues with food absorption? If your doctor has told you that you have problems absorbing certain vitamins and minerals and suggests supplements, you may consider if you're also having difficulty absorbing B vitamins

- Certain weight loss surgeries (stomach stints) and drugs may also interfere with B vitamin absorption.

- If you are over age 50 you may develop age-related vitamin deficiencies. Some around this age even opt to begin getting B12 shots at the doctor.

- Finally, if your diet is very poor in general, a deficiency may occur. If you're not a vegetarian, then ensure you are eating proper amounts of "real" meat. Fast food and other dubious sources do not count.

Quick B12 Boosts

One of the best ways to get a quick infusion of B vitamins is through liver. One serving of liver contains over 1,000% of your daily dosage of B12. Next are dairy products, including cheeses and eggs. Finally, one vegan option to consider is to try some concentrated yeast spreads, labeled Marmite in the UK and Vegemite in Australia, with either brand importable to the States.

---

[7] http://www.health.harvard.edu/blog/vitamin-b12-deficiency-can-be-sneaky-harmful-201301105780

These products are not always enjoyed (the old saying goes "you either love Marmite or hate Marmite") but they present a good option for vegans who want a natural source of B vitamins that does not come from dairy or meat. It is best served spread as a thin layer on whole wheat toast. The taste is very savory and a bit salty, and is usually enjoyed by anybody who likes strong flavors.

Vegetables

While B12 is acquired through supplementation, meat or dairy—B6 is also needed in your diet to ensure optimal health and to decrease the chance of mood disorders. A B6 deficiency is usually caused by not eating enough vegetables. To ensure you're getting enough B6, stock up on leafy greens at the store. One of the best sources, and my favorite "super food" is kale, which in addition to B vitamins contains large amounts of other nutrients. Fresh kale in your diet on a daily basis may help with numerous other deficiencies or health problems, as well.

The Importance of Maintaining Balanced Meals

Another contributor to mood health, and possible culprit of depression, is an imbalanced, poorly regulated diet. Nutritionists stress the importance of eating a balanced, full breakfast. Skipping meals or not making careful meal choices can lead to various ill effects, including anxiety, low energy levels, and mood swings, all of which can be mistaken for—or act as a precursor—to depression.

When I say "balanced" meals, what I mean is regulating intake of protein to carbohydrates, ensuring a proper amount of food is eaten per day without skipping meals, maintaining sources of green vegetables, and eliminating the greasy, unhealthy food that leaks into our diets through fast food and the diets of convenience.

To provide an example, let's take a worst case example: *Dunkin' Doughnuts Bob*

Bob is a busy guy. He works as a data entry specialist for a medical firm, a job that requires keeping the energy levels high through synthetic stimuli—namely sugar and caffeine, lest he fall asleep on the job. In the morning, before work, he'll eat two plain cake doughnuts and a cup of sugary coffee. This, he rationalizes, gives him the energy fix needed for the rest of the day's work.

By 9 AM he's at work, plugging away. However, by around 12:00 he notices a familiar feeling—*lethargy and fatigue*. All of those hard to metabolize simple carbohydrates has resulted in a condition known as reactive hypoglycemia. This is the result of the rapid increase and subsequent decline of blood sugar in the body caused by eating high sugar foods like white cake. This is coupled with a secondary chemical after-effect of the caffeine, where energetic highs are often followed by remedial lows. Combined together, by lunch-time Bob is a mess.

Bob, however, has learned that resupplying the caffeine and sugar chemicals seems to counteract the temporary tipping points. So for lunch he eats a slice of pizza, a sugary coke, and later followed by a cup of coffee. He's back to "normal again". By 5:00 he's leaving work, but on the drive home he feels like he's going to drive off the edge of the road.

He returns home, completely spent of energy. He spends the rest of his evening vegging out on the couch, way more drained than he should be. As a result of periodically going unconscious, he totally skips dinner. By 11 PM, he realizes he needs to eat something else, so he munches on a bag of Kettle Chips for 5 minutes, then passes out in his bedroom to begin another day of it. Now as Bob sleeps, his body is confused by skipping the meal, it's still trying to rapidly process all of the glucose he keeps consuming, and he's likely dehydrated as well, as his only sources of fluids all day came in the form of caffeine infused drinks that barely provided any actual hydration, as caffeine has a dehydrating effect. As a result of the dehydration, Bob wakes up the next morning feeling hungover. "That's odd," he thinks. "I didn't even drink anything last night."

A lifestyle like Bob's is a ticket to various health disorders, from diabetes, cancer to most immediately—*depression*. The sugar and caffeine crashes he experiences throughout the day will continually alter his mood. His inability to eat consistent meals keeps him energy deficient when he should be metabolizing and fueling his brain, and further, his lack of green vegetables and omega fatty acids is probably depriving him of the amino acids and B vitamins that he needs to prevent the onset of various mood and neurological disorders.

It would then come as no surprise when Bob begins suffering from symptoms of depression. He no longer has much motivation to go to work, he loses touch with his friends and family members, begins to neglect personal maintenance, his apartment falls into disrepair, and he even starts to show signs of obesity and premature aging. Eventually, upon the encouragement of family, Bob goes to see a doctor. The doctor quickly prescribes him antidepressants, which Bob adds to his cocktail of morning chemicals like white sugar and caffeine. At no point does the doctor ask Bob about his lifestyle choices or what he's eating. Because the doctor did not mention it, Bob assumes to keep everything at the status quo, and believes his depression is a combination of unrelated factors—possibly a chemical imbalance, of which a lifetime supply of expensive, toxic pharmaceuticals is the only cure.

What Bob Should Do

Bob's habits are, undoubtedly, a mild (or even moderate) form of addiction. The first most important thing is for Bob to connect the dots together that his depressive symptoms and mood swings are directly the result of his lifestyle and eating choices. It's not until he fully realizes this will he have the motivation to make a change, because then he could equate dietary change with the possibility of fixing his lousy feelings, which will give him a strong enough incentive to do something about it.

Bob should immediately:

- Begin shopping at a grocery store and preparing meals. Going to *Dunkin' Doughnuts* because of the convenience is dangerous. When his energy levels return, he won't need to continue fast food, as he only eats there to avoid being late for work when he doesn't have the energy to get out of bed.

- Eliminate breakfasts that are high on simple carbs (glucose). Immediately replace them with kale omelets, which will provide a great source of B vitamins, amino acids, and protein, with perhaps a slice of whole wheat toast for enough *good carb*s to give him real energy. If he is not a vegetarian, adding chicken to the omelet will increase his B12 and tryptophan levels and provide more protein.

- Begin cutting back on the coffee, as the caffeine may be further hurting his mood. To wean off it, he should start switching to green tea, which can still provide an adequate caffeine boost, but with the addition of antioxidants and other health benefits of tea.

- To drink, he should begin switching to water, vegetable juices, unsweetened iced teas or fruit infused waters. He should completely eliminate all forms of soft drinks from his life.

- Bob should try some exercise. He may not like exercise, so he should think about doing something he likes to do, like tennis or football matches every couple of days, to at least get some sunlight (serotonin) and cardio work. (For more about good exercise habits, see my main book <u>30 Days to Amazing Health</u>).

- Bob should prepare some of his own meals in a cooler and bring them to work to avoid the bad choices at his workplace cafeteria, which probably includes a lot of French fries, chicken nuggets, and pizza. He should load up on things like whole wheat tuna sandwiches with kale and fresh avocados.

- Bob should devote some serious time to cleaning up his apartment. Something as simple as a messy bed can have a psychological impact that can lower your sense of well-being, and that old stack of magazines and newspapers in the corner isn't helping, either

- Finally, Bob should learn to eliminate stress through some meditation. He can even make his space more conducive to those "good vibes" by incorporating some incense or maybe a pleasant picture on the wall.

Overeating

Just as skipping meals can alter your mood, so can eating too much, which sometimes even occurs as a symptom of depression; as sufferers seek an easy solution to quell their bad feelings by eating a tub of mac & cheese.

While overeating can be a psychological symptom, it can also be a cause. Unfortunately, the food industry is often designed to manipulate eaters into eating more, thus *buying more*. One way this is done is through high fructose corn syrup. Despite what the corn lobby would have you believe, HFCS really is quite bad for you. A study done at the University of Pennsylvania found that fructose does not suppress a hunger hormone known as ghrelin the same way that table sugar does. This means food sweetened by HFCS may not satisfy your hunger, which will encourage you to eat larger and larger portions. This can, of course, lead to various health problems, including obesity, food addiction and ultimately depression.

This study should also raise some warning bells about fructose in general. While fruit is part of a balanced diet, especially for the healthy antioxidants in berries and vitamins like C in citrus, some people overdo fruit consumption, and the fructose that comes with it. This is especially a problem with genetically modified farming, where GMO fruits may contain even larger amounts of fructose than nature would have allowed. The fructose can then lead to overeating and out of control glucose levels.

Portion sizes can also be manipulated to maximal effect. Fast food French fries, for instance, are hollow inside, which is to minimize production costs and prevent eaters from feeling full (and it's no surprise, the fries are also coated with HFCS solutions to further prevent feelings of hunger while addicting the eater to the high sugar content). Any current or former French fry eater may recall how no amount of those things ever satiate your cravings!

The bottom line? Stay vigilant and beware of commercially produced food. Stay away from golden arches, and prepare your own meals as much as you can, using fresh ingredients. And, always check the ingredients labels before you buy. If there's HFCS present, throw it out!

An Unscientific Observation

Do you ever notice eating something really bad makes you feel "yucky"? As an example, fast food. My anti fast-food diet regulations were, in the past, not as strict as they are today. A taco bell greasy ques*athingy* would usually taste kind-of good at the time, and about 30 minutes later I just wouldn't feel completely right. Most of the time it would just pass through my system, but if I were unlucky (and the cook decided not to wear his gloves or wash his hands), it could later cause gastro problems.

Our health is interconnected between many different areas, much as our cells—billions of tiny creatures—are all connected to create one complete organism. In an interconnected whole, all it takes is for one bad link on the chain to cause effects everywhere else. Consuming a greasy McWhattheheckkdidijusteat could immediately jeopardize your entire system, if only in a small way. This leads to your body sending various signals to *stop doing that.*

This is maybe why eating food that is filled with: chemicals, preservatives, poor hygienic standards, trans fat, deep fried residues, gummy simple carbs (white cake), high fructose corn syrup and other nutritional "no no's" makes us just generally feel *bad* all over.

And when you feel bad, you lose sync with your emotions. If you're already simply trudging through the day with low energy levels and feelings of unease, imagine how much worse it is when you're delivered bad news at work or in your personal life, or when something small happens like someone steals your parking space. Whatever bad things happen to you suddenly become exponentially worse.

And that is probably the most impactful way that bad food causes depression. There's no denying now that what you eat is going to determine your mood and well-being, so hopefully this is good enough motivation for you to start making these necessary lifestyle changes.

Chapter Three – Supplemental Pill Strategies

While supplements are generally best consumed via digested form in the foods we eat, to treat depression specifically, sometimes isolated vitamins and minerals can have a strong positive effect. Do keep in mind before beginning any kind of supplemental regiment, talk to a doctor first. Many of us have strange reactions to various plants and minerals; including even dangerous allergies or hazardous reactions to other medications you may be taking.

St. John's Wort

St. John's Wort, also known as the plant *Hypericum perforatum*, has long been marketed as a "natural anti-depressant". The herb appears to regulate your body's serotonin levels, and there is scientific data to support taking it if you're a sufferer of depression. Unlike other vitamins or herbs, St. John's Wort is particularly potent and it does not take long for mood alterations to occur.

According to Klaus Linde, from the Center for Complimentary Medicine in Munich: "Overall, we found that the St. John's wort extracts tested in the trials were superior to placebos and as effective as standard antidepressants, with fewer side effects."[8].

According to the Cochraine study, published in 2008, St. John's Wort compared favorably to other anti-depression remedies among a group of 5,489 patients, with fewer patients ending their treatment early as a result of fewer side-effects as compared to pharmaceutical counterparts.

However, just because St. John's Wort is "natural", users need to beware of adverse health effects. According to a report by the National Center for Complimentary and Integrative Health, St.

---

[8] http://www.sciencedaily.com/releases/2008/10/081007192435.htm

John's Wort can pose serious side-effects when taken with other supplements or pharmaceuticals, including a sudden rise of serotonin levels that can become dangerous or even fatal[9].

This is why, before beginning St. John's Wort treatment, you should speak to a professional—and most importantly, not be currently taking any other supplements or pharmaceuticals, at least until you speak to an expert first.

Otherwise, this herb could be a very useful alternative treatment, to obtain the effects of anti-depressants without the chemical side-effects.

Vitamin D

Vitamin D can be supplemented into your diet in pill or liquid form, or increased in your diet through additional milk and dairy consumption, although experts warn that simply digesting vitamin D rich foods is not enough, and proper vitamin D levels require either supplements and / or the primary source; which is exposure of your bare skin to sunlight. If depression is an issue for you, then vitamin D cannot be forgotten about, as studies have linked deficiencies in D directly to the common symptoms of depression[10]. Scientists are not entirely sure why the vitamin affects mood, but studies have found that brain cells appear to contain receptors specifically designed to function with D. Receptors are like "nodules" where chemicals attach to give a cell instructions to perform actions like division. Apparently, one such unknown function includes vitamin D, and it's thought it may relate to chemical balance or the brain's intercellular communication abilities. This may explain why a lack of the vitamin seems to cause a type of cognitive breakdown.

Vitamin D is another one of those vitamins that must be handled cautiously and with moderation. Excess amounts of supplementation can lead to a serious condition called hypervitamonisis D, which can include cognitive disabilities. Basically, too little D can lead to mood

---

[9] https://nccih.nih.gov/health/stjohnswort/sjw-and-depression.htm
[10] http://www.vitasearch.com/get-clp-summary/40584

and mental dysfunction, and too much can create almost the exact same effect. Your brain requires a delicate balance.

Magnesium

Another drawback to the Western diet is the depletion of certain essential minerals through the erosion caused by our favorite chemicals: caffeine, sugar, alcohol and cortisol (stress hormones). One such mineral that we lose is magnesium.

Magnesium is an extremely important human building block. It is the counter ion for calcium and potassium in muscle cells, which means a lack of magnesium can cause calcium related side-effects like cramping, leading up to the most severe side-effect of depletion: sudden heart failure and death. In other words, it would be wise to maintain the RDV of Magnesium.

In addition, there is some heavy speculation that magnesium has a big effect on mood and depression. There have been private, independent studies that have demonstrated a "major" positive effect on mood by increasing magnesium levels. An extensive report, carried out by George and Karen Eby and published in the Medical Hypotheses journal, discusses how 70% of adults lack proper amounts of magnesium, and that stress—with it's ability to reduce magnesium, creates a type of "vicious cycle" of magnesium depletion, leading to more stress, thus leading to further deficiency[11]. The article traces magnesium and depression studies as far back as the 1920s, when it was used as an effective home remedy, up to more recent studies where simple 200mg increases of magnesium would apparently result in patients experiencing not only a decrease in depression, but also increased IQ and short-term memory abilities.

Although magnesium is not fully understood, and more clinical studies need to be carried out, it seems likely that it plays yet another role in brain circuitry and health.

---

[11] http://george-eby-research.com/html/magnesium-for-depression.pdf

Vitamin C

Our bodies, health and minds require equilibrium, and throwing this off center can lead to depression. One stabilizer that we require a constant source of is vitamin C. This vitamin acts as a binding support agent for the collagen and elastin that literally holds us together. This is why a vitamin C deficiency, known as scurvy, can result in loosening of gums and other parts of the skin, as well as jaundice (skin yellowing).

In addition, vitamin C plays important parts in mood and depression. According to a recent study among elderly patients, even mild vitamin C deficiencies were linked to mood problems and depression[12]. It is believed that the deficiency causes a lower level of neurotransmitters, and where there is more hindered communication among brain cells, there is a greater likelihood for mood disorders to develop. There is also ongoing research that links vitamin C with lower stress.

Your body cannot use more than 1,000 mg of vitamin C in a given dose, so it's not recommended to supplement more than this amount. By taking 1,000 mg of C per day, however, you will experience multiple health benefits, including improved heart health and hopefully a decreased chance for depression.

SAM-E

SAM-E, otherwise known as Ademetionine, Adenosylmethionine, Adénosylméthionine (I prefer the shorter version), is a very interesting supplement I've discovered recently. This is a molecule that circulates in the blood naturally, but has been chemically formulated in a lab. It works as a "methyl donor", which means that it adds methyl to other molecules, serving the purpose of fixing and maintaining metabolic processes. The theory surrounding SAM-E is that certain medical conditions are associated with a lack of SAM-E circulation, and when SAM-E levels drop, a person becomes

---

[12] http://www.ncbi.nlm.nih.gov/pubmed/20808095

predisposed to conditions like osteoarthritis, diabetes, and depression. Restoring SAM-E levels to a normal or increased rate may then lessen these diseases.

SAM-E is an interesting pill that lies somewhere in-between a natural supplement and a chemical pharmaceutical, but it certainly does not host the side-effects of normal drugs. In addition, it has been considered as a beneficial side-pill to take alongside anti-depressants, and is recommended by some doctors for this purpose. However, more research needs to be done about the safety of SAM-E supplementation, especially when mixed with other drugs / supplements. A 2010 study by the American Journal of Psychiatry provided 800mg of SAM-E to depression patients in conjunction with medications; and found an improvement by comparison to a placebo[13].

Studies have shown 800-1600 mg daily doses of SAM-E to be almost as effective as medications prescribed for osteoarthritis, as well as depression. This makes the pill a potentially very effective depression treatment, although the exact nature of how it works remains somewhat elusive.

I think it remains a very promising new supplement that should be taken seriously by anyone who suffers from depression.

GABA

The long name for this supplement is Gamma-aminobutyric acid. This is an amino acid neurotransmitter that has been synthesized as a component of many of the pharmaceutical anti-depressants on the market today.

GABA acts as a nerve transmission inhibitor. What these do is essentially help a person to regulate the signals coming through the brain, preventing the types of nervous overloads that are present among people with depression or anxiety disorders. In fact, many

---

[13] http://ajp.psychiatryonline.org/doi/abs/10.1176/appi.ajp.2009.09081198

nervous conditions are related to the presence (or non-presence) of GABA; for instance, caffeine inhibits GABA release, and it's no surprise that too much caffeine makes us feel "jittery".

GABA is part of a very interesting area of research that could be shedding light on a host of different mental disorders. For instance, researchers have discovered that improper amounts of GABA could be the culprit behind bipolar disorder, and a potential major factor in many types of depression.[14]

The idea of taking the GABA molecules in their raw form is to bypass the chemically synthetic version; and inhibit our nerves without the nasty side-effects. However, the problem with this is that pharmaceuticals are designed to directly carry a chemical past the blood-brain barrier. Taking these molecules raw means there is no function for the GABA to begin joining with your other neural amino acids. And so, according to doctors and pharmacists, it's probably a time waster, and health experts would suggest to find a supplement that implements more GABA through absorption of a different nutrient (like theanine).

Then again, taking GABA supplements have shown some positive effect among users. So, is there some type of hidden function present that scientists don't know? That might be up to you to find out, as taking the supplement is certainly safer to "experiment" with than taking a drug. That being said, side-effects have still been reported; including neural changes like tingling sensations and rapid heart-beat (which poses the question; if there are side-effects that seem to correlate with an increase of GABA in the brain, then wouldn't that mean it's working?).

GABA is not a completely clear area, to be sure. However, if you're looking to try something different, it may be worth checking out. Both natural and isolated forms of the amino acid are available in pill form.

---

[14] Petty F, Kramer GL, Fulton M, Moeller FG, Rush AJ. Low plasma GABA is a trait-like marker for bipolar illness. Neuropsychopharmacology. 1993 Sep;9(2):125-32.

Fish Oil

In the last chapter, I discussed the importance of omega-3 fatty acids for brain health, and how there is a lot of research pointing to good fats as the essential building blocks of a healthy brain. As a result, many depression experts suggest to begin supplementing with fish oil capsules to get that extra omega-3 boost that likely everyone needs.

I personally feel it's a better idea to consume your omega-3 versus use pills. Dietitians often say that it's wiser to absorb nutrients like these through food, as it has a higher chance of being metabolized throughout your body, versus in a liquid gel-cap form, which may just flush right out. However, research seems to vary on this topic and there are other nutritionists who swear by the capsule-form.

Aside from taking capsules, you can also get a nice source of fish oil the "real way" by buying marinated sardines in oil. Combine that with some avocado and you'll have a great little omega-3 fatty acid diet going!

Theanine

L-Theanine is amino acid derivative taken from green tea. The function of this supplement relates to the GABA amino acid chain that I discussed earlier. Theanine, according to some research, appears to promote GABA production in the brain, which (as we've learned) means a greater inhibition of nerve firings, acting as a type of natural anti-depressant.

Theanine is also a well-known cure dating back thousands of years, as the Chinese have been drinking tea for as long as humans have been making cups. Studies in Japan have shown an improvement of sleep quality as well as mood as a result of 200mg of theanine consumption. This may explain the subtly relaxing benefit of many types of teas.

The concentrated variety is suggested to be taken in the 200mg to 300mg range; otherwise you can enjoy the benefits by simply implementing more tea into your diet. Green tea is the best source, but even normal teas may have some level of theanine as well as other good nutrients, like antioxidants.

Valerian Root

Traditionally, valerian root has been administered for centuries for various ills, including: stomach cramps, insomnia, anxiety, and stress. The reason that it appears to have some basis in soothing nerves relates to an ability to affect neurotransmitters (possibly affecting amino-acids, like GABA). Although the function and effectiveness is not entirely understood or known, many swear by valerian pills or teas to help get through the day.

Because the function isn't entirely known, it's not recommended to take valerian with prescription pills or other supplements before first speaking to a doctor. And, some side effects have been reported where valerian actually promotes the symptom it's supposed to cure; for instance causing insomnia among those trying to sleep.

Add valerian to your anti-depression arsenal with a little bit of caution, but it's definitely worth trying out. Everybody's bodies are different, and certainly some of us react more favorably to certain supplements than others.

5-HTP

Before we discussed the benefits of tryptophan, found in meats like poultry and certain vegetables. What some are unaware of, however, is that scientists have isolated the actual chemical property that tryptophan creates in the brain, known as 5-HTP, which raises your serotonin levels. Some studies have shown that 5-HTP can be used effectively to treat mild to moderate depression, with doses of 5-HTP matching the effectiveness of the pharmaceutical antidepressant known as Luvox[15].

The process of isolation is actually done through natural ingredients. 5-HTP has been found in a pure form in the seeds of an African plant called Griffonia simplicifolia. It has since been extracted and turned into a supplement that can be taken in pill form, usually in-between 100 and 300 mg per dose, with a recommended dosage of three times per day.

As with many supplements, 5-HTP has variables to consider. Firstly, commercial 5-HTP was widely publicized in the late 1980s and early 1990s for containing impurities that led to fatal occurrences of a disease known as eosinophilia myalgia syndrome—a neurological condition involving over-production of white blood cells. It's believed this was the result of over-engineered 5-HTP from an aggressive Japanese manufacturer. Today, most 5-HTP supplements list they are free of the contaminant that was reported as "Peak X".

In addition, 5-HTP has been under scrutiny by some reports that have said that as a supplement it could actually worsen depression symptoms[16]. As with many supplements or chemicals that interfere with or increase serotonin levels, it seems there is a fine balancing act to perform, as boosting serotonin too much yields the exact opposite of the desired results, which is why it's wisest to consult first with a doctor.

Putting it All Together: What's Right For You?

The wrong approach to supplements (and also the expensive approach) is the shotgun method; to buy up large amounts of these and start popping pills hoping your depression will go away. As you may have noticed from the warnings I've attached to these, there are serious considerations to think about; from how these affect other medications and supplements, to the function of a specific supplement and if it is the right measure for your specific condition. For instance, it would be unwise to take two different supplements

---

[15] http://umm.edu/health/medical/altmed/supplement/5hydroxytryptophan-5htp
[16] http://www.ncbi.nlm.nih.gov/pmc/articles/PMC3415362/#!po=65.3846

that boost serotonin levels, as this could put you in danger of a serotonin disorder which could actually magnify your depression symptoms.

The wisest option is to find an open-minded doctor—one who's not bias against non-pharmaceutical alternatives—and figure out what you should take. You may even be subject to some tests to discover if there are any vitamins or minerals specifically that you might deficient in, and then the supplements could directly target the source of your symptoms.

Short of that, the best strategy is to combine the foods listed in the first chapter with one or two supplements from this chapter, carefully selected and taken with consideration and caution. In addition, implement large amounts of exercise with healthy amounts of sunlight, and apply some of the techniques we'll be going over in the next chapter. Combining all of this together will, I feel, provide a very good chance of nullifying your depression.

Chapter Four – Purely Holistic Depression Cures

Many of the techniques we've covered so far, even through natural therapies, ultimately relate to the chemical side of depression. But, to think of depression as much more than these mechanistic principles, we need to explore topics like nature, our social lives, negative energies, and our general lifestyles. It's only after we achieve a level of harmony with our diet, environment, chemicals, lifestyle and philosophy that we can be sure that depression will be eliminated, and stay gone.

The following are the best strategies I can devise, in no particular order, to kick depression out of your life:

Technique 1: Get Back in Touch With Nature

Parks, mountains, forests, beaches—these are all outdoor activities you can enjoy, with no requirement to do anything other than simply be present in these environments and soak up the fresh air. However, don't take my word for it. In fact, according to a study published in the journal of Epidemiology and Community Health, the prevalence of clusters of disease are significantly reduced in environments with greater green space in a 1km radius, with specific implications in regard to depression and anxiety related conditions[17].

What this means is that if you're confined to a working environment in the inner-city, then it becomes an imperative to reconnect with nature. It seems to be something that our bodies simply crave, as historically the advent of big, concrete vertical slabs, smog and roads is a very new phenomenon, and the human being is not adapted to live under these conditions.

---

[17] http://jech.bmj.com/content/63/12/967.short

In addition, it also fulfills the need for moderate (healthy) amounts of sunlight, in-order to regulate serotonin and vitamin D levels.

There are ways, of course, to implement this into a lifestyle or a job. Hobbies like gardening and hiking provide a convenient way to get your sunlight and your dose of green. And, more "comprehensive" steps could also be implemented; for instance, one person I know gave up her office job to become a type of shepherd in the countryside for a non-profit organization that helps animals. Another person I know began working exclusively online, while selling his old home to move the family to just outside the city limits to the countryside, in an eco-sustainable house.

The very least you can do is make a habit to go to your local park every now and then. It could be where you exercise. Do it when the sun is out, and practice this as a form of meditation and relaxation.

Technique 2: Charity

Do not underestimate the powerful potential of giving back to the world! Not every cause of depression is physiological and chemical. We are an infinitely complex web of different psychological states, which ranges from reliving past traumas to obsessing about the future, to even completely irrational but very negative states of mind about the world and the people in it (otherwise known as cynicism).

There is no immediate cure for negativity, but there is one technique that comes pretty close—giving back to people. You can do it in small ways (a smile) or big ways (a check to an honest organization), or just in a routine way (volunteering weekly to something meaningful). The point is that charity is a special type of work that basically removes the ego from the picture. While most of the time we are mostly concerned with what we are going to get back in return for our work, when you are doing something solely for others then you have a different measurement of success.

I do believe a cause of depression is when a person has too much focus on the self and not enough on others. This can become a lifestyle where all that a person knows how to do is worry about the acquisition of things like wealth and respect. Flaws and minor problems in life can start to seem much worse when you are framing everything in the context of your self-worth.

Charity is one way around this. If you do not have the time or money to do anything drastic, just consider how you can help people around you in small ways on a day to day basis.

Technique 3: Meditation and Visualizations

You might be used to seeing my suggestions for meditation and visualization that I include in most of my books. The reason is because this remains a key to a healthy lifestyle, and science agrees as increasing research in fields like epigenetics and the placebo effect shows how closely related the mind and body are. Simply thinking about and focusing on something enough seems to make it a reality, at least as far as our bodies and our health is concerned.

A big part of battling depression is figuring out what is going wrong with your thoughts on an internal level. Traditionally, this is what psychotherapy seeks to help with. You can assist this process by first relaxing your body, relaxing your mind, and then engaging with specific visualizations that target areas of stress, anxiety or negativity.

Calm your environment. Dim lights. Shut off distractions, so turn off your phone. Take some time-out from your kids if you have any. Light incense or play some relaxing music. Sit in a comfortable chair. Focus on breathing for 10 minutes. When this is done, ask yourself how you are feeling inside. Reflect on the day, and consider where you are feeling anxiety and what aspects of your daily routine are causing them.

If you find yourself feeling deficient in some area, for instance a belief that you are "not good enough" at a task in your job, that you are not a good spouse, that you are not attractive, or any other negative mindset, you must then create a visualization that is tuned to the opposite direction.

For instance: *"I excel at that area of my job. I am a great spouse and always becoming better. Everyone feels I am attractive and charming."*

It's not enough to repeat these visualizations once, but now you must exercise them constantly, including first thing in the morning when you wake up. You must also learn to *feel* what your words are. It's not enough to repeat something, but you must place yourself deeply within that context.

Technique 4: Sleep

A lack of sleep can lead to metabolic issues, a weakened immune system, and mood disorders. Sleep is the time when your body refuels, and neglecting it can have disastrous results. All too often, however, busy people forget that a minimal of 8 hours of sleep per night is required for an energetic, healthy lifestyle. And, if you have been on a low-sleep schedule for a long time, you may want to consider upping it to 9-10 hours a night as you transition into a more restful lifestyle.

It never stops amazing me when people I know begin discussing symptoms like depression, anxiety, eating disorders, digestive disorders, etc—and I find out they are sleeping about 4 hours per night! I hear justifications about this, and in university days the myth would perpetuate of "Well, I'm young, so I can handle it!"

Even a young person who is not sleeping adequately is going to experience big problems. So, there really is no skipping it.

So how do you sleep more?

The answer really involves scheduling time. On a 9-5 work day, we may feel energized after our job, and we have a desire to stay up past bed time to keep unwinding a little longer, maybe watching our favorite TV shows or doing any manner of activities.

What you should do is instead focus on "slowing the pace" an hour before bed. If you go to sleep at 11 AM and wake up at 7, then begin breaking away from digital media by 10 PM. You can try something like the meditation and visualization exercise I spoke of in the last technique to finish your night. I'd avoid any kind of serious mental stimuli during this time, and this even includes novel reading.

One of the main reasons people experience insomnia is that their minds just won't shut off. This is often because they don't give themselves proper time to relax and unplug from stimuli first.

Technique 5: Aromatherapy

Aromatherapy is the use of essential oils to improve your mental state (mood) and health. It remains a viable technique to combat depression. The exact nature of how aromatherapy works remains speculative by scientists, who simply link certain fragrances with pleasant mood alterations. Aromatherapists, however, see it as a much more intricate topic that goes beyond the scents themselves.

There are several ways to implement essential oils:

- **Aerosols:** These will create a fragrance in your entire room. You can find aerosol formulations of most essential oils.
- **Diffusion:** This is done via a diffusion machine, which blends a scent into the entire room over time, keeping the fragrance sustained in the air.
- **Baths:** Salts and oils can be implemented into the bathtub to create the aromatherapeutic effect.
- **Massage:** Many spas also implement aromatherapy and essential oils into massage treatments.

For depression, aromatherapists recommend the following essential oils:

- Basil
- Bergamot
- Clary Sage
- Geranium
- Jasmine
- Neroli
- Petitgrain
- Sandalwood
- Ylang-Ylang

When getting involved with aromatherapy, consider first if you may have any allergic reactions to the oils in question, Test first by applying small amounts, and ensuring there are no adverse effects before moving on with a larger amount.

Aromatherapy is effective when implementing it with other practices, like meditation.

Technique 6: Career Overhaul

There's no way to put this mildly: some jobs lead to depression. And, it's not worth it. It will never be worth it. We spend a large chunk—usually more than half—of our waking lives involved in some type of for-profit work activity. So, if this activity is not in harmony, I believe you will quickly experience mental suffering.

What makes a good job? Here is some wisdom to digest: it really has nothing to do with the activity itself, but the quality of your coworkers and the lifestyle that surrounds it. That simple! Your dream job could involve architecture, but how much would you enjoy a job at an architectural firm if your boss is a micromanager with severe bipolar disorder who also sexually harasses co-workers? Probably not so much.

Unfortunately, I believe toxic work environments are the standard and not the exception. You have to look to find somewhere that is a healthy environment, and it's usually not your first pick. I believe it really involves maturity among management. Somebody in charge of other people's livelihood must have good leadership skills, sensibilities, and a level of empathy. If management does not possess these things, morale will drop, workers get depressed, and things slowly fall to pieces.

Depression can also occur if you know for a fact you're not living up to your full potential. If you work as a waitress and you are depressed about the mindless grind and rude customers you experience every day, then why the heck are you still doing it? Usually the answer is fear. We fear changing things, and the unknown. We believe resigning means we'll have no other options, and end up scrounging in dumpsters.

Unless you are living in a less-than-developing-country, this won't happen to you. And even if you are in a country with a poor economy, you'll still probably be OK and find a better opportunity. Once you become pro-active and you start thinking about how you can best offer your real talents to the workplace, doors will open for you and you'll be extremely happy that you decided to be done with serving coffee and juggling plates of omelets.

A trickier situation is if your job pays very well, also known as the infamous "Golden Handcuffs". You may work at a firm and be making a sizable, 6-figure income, with the only drawback being personal suffering and a degradation of your mental health. My answer again is simple: during your last days before you die, you won't be looking back and thinking "I'm sure glad I suffered another five years in that job I hated". If you really are unhappy, find a way to get out—because depression is not worth the paycheck.

Technique 7: Feng Shui

Practitioners of feng shui believe the placement of objects in a room affects the flow of qi—vital life force—which thus determines the amount of positive energy in an environment. Ancients took this concept very seriously. Chinese and Indian traditions blended together, and the city designs of many places in India actually follow these principles.

There is a substantial amount of evidence for the existence of qi (chi) energy, which can be found if you study the seemingly supernatural powers of certain monks and martial artists from regions like Tibet. If the Chinese have long believed that qi is sensitive to factors like the arrangements in a room, it may be worth listening to.

A more skeptical point of view would argue feng shui is just about the pleasing symmetry. Studies have shown certain symmetrical patterns create pleasure, compared to off-kilter arrangements that spread feelings of disharmony. As an example, a beautiful face has rather specific mathematical measurements, compared to an "ugly" face that lacks that same symmetrical composition.

Feng shui is typically performed by an expert who overlays a **bagua map** over the room schematics. The expert will then attempt to achieve a yin-yang balance of different elemental themes (according to Chinese tradition, different elemental powers act on each other either productively or destructively, for instance wood produces fire).

On the bagua grid, you will find 9 colors: black (career, office things), blue (skills and wisdom, books and your computer), green (family, plants and family photos), purple (signs of prosperity), red (fame and reputation, so things like awards and diplomas), pink (love and relationships, items paired together or family photos), white (creativity, which could mean artwork), gray (travel, souvenirs), yellow (health, symbols of health like statues).

The feng shui expert will attempt to then see that your home achieves a balance in all of these areas. From a psychological point of view, a home may not feel very much like something that is "yours" unless there is a balance of different aspects of your life: from your career, to reminders of your accomplishments in life, to symbols of family and loved ones. Without these components, your abode could become—for lack of a better word—depressing!

So, if you are not interested in paying hundreds to a feng shui consultant, you can at least think about balancing the 9 "colors" in your home and seeing how this improves your mood. In addition, consider ensuring your environment remains positive and uplifting by consistently cleaning, disposing of refuse, keeping the beds tidy, and letting in more sunlight from various corners. The addition of potted plants can also help with this, as it brings a bit of "life" into your environment.

Technique 8: Increase Social Activities

Humans are social creatures and we are *meant* to have friends and family around. Is it any surprise, as I mentioned at the very beginning of this book, that cultures outside of America have depression rates cut in half or less? I believe this is because the United States, and probably countries like Canada and Australia as well, are extremely individualistic to a fault. The "every man for himself" state of mind seems to imprint itself energetically on the people, and many would prefer to do things like stay at home and watch TV or YouTube instead of spending time with real people. This is in contrast to communal / family cultures found all around the world, where neighbors and friends are sharing wine on a nightly basis.

I find it no surprise then that my fellow Americans are sometimes longing for social contact, without even realizing it. Putting on dinner parties, mixers and daytime activities with friends and neighbors often draws people who start looking forward to nothing else but those things all week long. Yes, it's quite easy to become a social "queen bee" if you are the one who takes the initiative to do it.

As so many people seem to be starved for social attention, I am guessing that you might be, also. Isolation is definitely a cause for depression, and it could be the factor in your life that you're forgetting about.

So, just start focusing on more social activities. One great way I discovered to meet people is to join a community college class. Or start attending or even joining sports matches, like tennis. Or, start hosting get-togethers (dinner, cocktail parties, etc). One person I know even started creating her own art gallery shows—how's that for a great opportunity to meet people?

Technique 9: Take Care of an Animal

Please note that I am not suggesting to become a "crazy cat lady" as a means to alleviate depression—although I've certainly seen this happen to people on more than one occasion. The reason people do things like buy cats is because, clearly, it works. Nothing like having a little furry creature running around who loves you unconditionally to pick your spirits up.

Obviously, take some care before deciding to raise up a living creature. If your depression is severe, it might not be such a good idea—as if you are not in a position where you can take care of yourself, it would not be wise to try and take care of another living creature. Buying a kitten is probably a good solution if your symptoms are milder.

If you don't want the responsibility (and sense of attachment) that may come with an animal like a dog or a cat, you could even do something as simple as buying some fish and a small tank. It might sound silly, but just the act of taking care of other living creatures— even ones as simple as fish—can have a very positive effect on you.

Technique 10: Take a Long Vacation / Adventure

Your problems in life may seem very near to you right now, but how badly would they affect you when you are hiking with a guide through the wilderness of Mongolia? Okay, this is a slightly extreme example, but the point remains that if you do something that completely shakes up your world—you may find your old problems melt away and new unimaginable possibilities open up for you.

So, where to go? There are many possibilities. Common destinations like West Europe or Caribbean islands can be very expensive and crowded, so if you want to have a mind-expanding experience that will stay with you for a long time, I'd suggest looking elsewhere on the map. A couple I knew went on an extended trip in Morocco which included camel rides in the desert—pretty amazing. You could also go to an off-the-beaten-map country like Armenia, Serbia or somewhere in Central Asia, like Kazakhstan. The possibilities are endless, and it's not as expensive as you think!

You may be wondering how one can afford something like this, and the best solution is sometimes to have a yard sale and begin liquidating all of the things you don't want or need anymore out of your life, while at the same time saving money for an epic vacation. This by itself actually has a therapeutic effect, because in life it is very often true that there is no link between material possessions and happiness. In fact a lot of times, the exact opposite is true. Getting rid of that old sofa for $25 may also mean purging the bad memories that went with it.

When you're done with the yard sale—and after you're back from your adventures abroad, you may find a more Spartan living space will help to clear your mind. There is something about having a stack of old magazines from the 1990s stacked high on an old stained coffee table that just really makes the mood more depressing. If you have a tendency to accumulate junk, then it's all the more reason to take this approach.

Technique 11: Begin a Process of Eliminating Negative Influences

Let me ask you something: how badly are other people with damaged personalities intensifying the stress and pressure of your own life? Many times our lives get infiltrated by those people most of us are all too familiar with—sociopaths, controllers, or extremely negative and dark people. This can have a powerful residual effect on your life and send an otherwise healthy person into a downward vortex of depression. This situation can be compounded if you're forced to live with or interact with that person on a daily basis.

Examples include:

- A boss
- A spouse
- A parent
- A sibling
- A roommate

This is obviously a touchy subject because you can't just excommunicate some of these people from your life, *with the exception* of instances of actual abuse, in which case it's justified to seek things like divorces or restraining orders. Otherwise, if the negativity that you deal with is that subtle, under-the-skin type, you'll probably need to develop coping strategies first and foremost.

- For your boss, is there a way you can be transferred to another department where he or she is less active and on the prowl? Sometimes the best first strategy is avoidance.

- For a spouse, communication is key. If he or she is frequently negative and subjecting you to that energy, then it needs to be made apparent that your spouse must become aware of their actions and try to prevent it in the future.

- For parents, gauge their moods as best you can and try to promote better moods. If your mom is often negative with the exception of when she's eating, then maybe go out and buy her food a bit more often.

- For siblings; enact that personal boundary and give them some tough love. They'll appreciate it in the future.

- For problem roommates, short of getting a new one, enact a boundary like you would a sibling. If they start bringing you down, say "HAULT!" and change the topic in a new direction ("No, I DON'T want to gossip about your ex, thank you"). A bit of confrontation about these issues is better than allowing their negativity to get the best of you.

For anyone else—like not very close friends and mere casual acquaintances—get rid of them! The fewer dark and negative people in your life, the happier you will become, guaranteed!

Technique 12: Minimize Television and Media Consumption

Okay, so I am not one of those people who thinks it's good to live in a bubble. Some people are so afraid of negativity that they insulate themselves entirely from things like the news and current events. And then, to make matters even scarier, these same people will go out and vote!

The other extreme, though, are people (like my parents) who sit around watching the news constantly, and freaking out about things that are either exaggerated or would play no rational role in anyone's lives.

There is no grand conspiracy to use the news to keep the masses uninformed. There's no need for a conspiracy because it happens naturally as a result of profit-centric business models. Hype, sensationalism and even downright lies promote viewers and traffic, which means advertising revenue. It's an unfortunate thing.

So, when there's a minor tragedy, it is blown up into the worst thing ever, as this means keeping the shareholders happy. This can also happen maliciously, when an innocent person becomes a victim of the media, turning an embarrassment into a full-blown scandal.

All of this negativity can hurt us, so exercise caution when you get absorbed by any news story. Likewise, television and fiction can have very negative influences on us. See how you feel after you give up sensationalized news sources as well as very dark and grim fiction television.

What you can do is find a reliable source for fact-driven reporting with less hype. Personally, I like Al-Jazeera America, as this station seems to reliably produce high-quality broadcasts without the never-ending gossip and spin of companies like CNN.

Summing Everything Up

I strongly believe it's a mistake to take a linear direction in treating depression. We can't just assume that it's a simple occurrence that is treated with a pill or even a dietary change. Human psychology is complicated….It's so complicated, it may be one of the most complex phenomena in the universe. So how do we simply medicate it and expect results?

As we talk about in the beginning of this book, we must avoid those dark vortices that send us on spirals of negativity and ultimately depression. From the arrangement of how your room looks, to how much sleep you're getting, and the types of positive versus negative influences you have around you, all of these things can create a subtle but powerful impact on your psychological well-being.

Chapter Five – Philosophies For Depression and a Better Life

There are many techniques that make an effect on depressive illnesses, but one of the best long-term defense strategies is to build a solid life philosophy that will help you to handle life's tumults. I am not a philosopher or even a self-help coach, but these are just pointers that help me out and perhaps you will find benefit from, as well.

Finding the Moment

Eckhart Tolle's "Power of Now" series discusses the ability to transcend the worries of the past and the uncertainties of the future in-order to maintain a powerful, even transcendent focus on the immediate moment around you as it's unfolding, as he points out the illusionary nature of time itself.

What is it like to be truly present? Ask a pro basketball player or anybody else who performs an art or craft to perfection. However, their answer may sound very nebulous to you. "I just do it," they may say.

The reason is because there's no "thought" behind what they do, it happens during a flow-state. And, there's something even more powerful about this state: the fact that when we enter it, it seems like we enter a state of pure contentment! It seems our overactive minds are the things that really damage our happiness.

Ironically, it's the very act of overthinking about the future that sends us on the wrong course of direction where we may be susceptible to failure. The more we worry, the more likely that what we fear is going to come into reality. By contrast, the more we focus on the immediacy of "now" the more skilled we will become at virtually everything we do, and those problems we fear will be eliminated before our very eyes.

I believe a lot of times depression is attributed to a mental cycle that is *stuck on repeat*. We keep thinking about some idea over and over again, trying to understand it, preempt it or rationalize it. We also mistakenly believe that learning a skill or solving a problem requires mental gear grinding. Not so much.

The interesting thing about living in the *now* is that it's a mental philosophy that can be practiced with immediate noticeable results once you get the hang of it. And, to achieve it you don't even have to perform any lengthy meditation or visualization exercises. You could be driving in your car when you suddenly experience a total connection to the moment as it's happening, and the happiness that comes with that feeling.

I suggest to start actively training yourself to *not think* about the past or the future. Look around you and repeat the following: *Everything around me at this moment is everything that is, and nothing else is anything more than potential.*

Try this, and see what happens.

Finding a Higher Life Purpose

As I talked about at the very beginning of this book, to be depressed is to have a *compression* on your state of mind. If you're not living up to your real potential in life, it will feel like you're in a car compactor being slowly crushed to death! An example is if you take a passionate archaeologist and force her to work at *Burger King*. See how she'll feel after a few months of that!

Maybe the hard part is just finding whatever that calling might be, and then making a life out of it. Sometimes we don't even realize we're not following something else we're supposed to be doing, and therefore we don't even realize why it is we're depressed.

Another great thing about the "higher calling" strategy is that it makes other problems in your life feel a little bit impactful. To illustrate what I am saying, consider how extraordinary stresses happen to every single one of us. You don't really know what stress is like until something happens to you like you have a child who you find out has been born with a serious health problem. Or, you sit and watch a friend die. Many things like this will happen to all of us.

The powerful traumatic effect of these experiences won't go away, but if you have a higher calling in life—that won't go away, either. I like to think of some great filmmaker or playwright, somebody like William Shakespeare, or Oscar Wilde. Even when really bad things happen to these types of people, it will probably get channeled into some new work of art. In other words, the show goes on no matter what happens. And this is a really powerful way to deal with adversity. Aside from the arts, another example could be a mission in life to accomplish a goal or make the world a better place. While personal circumstances may cause stress or depression, the mission must continue forward and this can provide a person with the willpower and strength to keep going at all times.

Your Inner Child

Freudian psychology made the "inner child" concept enter our vernacular, and you may have heard terms before like "get in touch with your inner child" but what does this mean?

My interpretation (I am not a psychologist) is that when we are children we see the world from a perspective that is very care free and egoless. Into adulthood we get progressively more and more weighted down by life stresses as well as a sense of self-worth that is dependent on things like other people's approval

In other words, we no longer have the power to just be ourselves and enjoy life that happens around us. While little kids are lacking life lessons and wisdom, they are in some ways smarter than us emotionally. The way this applies to a philosophy is to begin tapping into that state of mind again.

The way I do it is when I feel a nagging sensation of shame if I am having too much fun, I immediately put it to rest. I don't know if there is a psychological term somewhere to describe this, but it's like when faced with life pressures, it becomes "shameful" or "wrong" to just let go, relax, or immerse into a hobby or passion.

For instance, when I was growing up one of my siblings really loved fantasy novels of various kinds. As she got older, she completely stopped having any interest in those types of things. However, I suspect it's not because she didn't like them anymore, but because society told her she was now supposed to be "grown up" and only care about adult responsibilities.

The irony here is that the adults who stay in touch with their inner child are usually the ones who are very successful, compared to adults who think only in terms of boring and rigid responsibilities. Even creative CEOs and entrepreneurs are this way, people like Virgin founder Richard Branson required a child-like enthusiasm and imagination to turn a small record store in England into a multinational with its own space travel division!

The takeaway point here is to look again at your hobbies and interests as a child and get back in touch with the things you enjoy, even if those things seem kind of "silly". The odds are those behaviors are closer to your real authentic self than the version of you who works in an office all day.

Time to Party and Laugh

I worry about people who don't party. Earlier, I mentioned how many other cultures have much lower depression rates it seems than the United States. It's no surprise then that some of the cultures in question have implemented parties and social gatherings into their day-to-day. As an example, it's customary for Italians to take long work breaks and crack open the wine in the middle of the day. While I don't condone so much alcohol, it sure is nice when you have socially enjoyable moments to look forward to every day.

As for laughter, the saying "laughter is the best medicine" has literal ramifications, with studies that have shown disease reduction and laughter being connected. I often speak of the intense power of the mind over the body, and it's no surprise that during its most lighthearted moments that the body seems to be most capable of healing itself.

There is a little bit of shame associated in Western culture with "partying", fun, and merriment, and this is what I believe we need to be very aware of. Just as there is shame around behaving through your inner child, there is a sense that if you're not working constantly, you're not "earning your keep", and taking time off to enjoy yourself is therefore a sign of some kind of laziness.

"I work 70 hours a week," some people say. "I don't have time for any of that."

It's very important to change your paradigm in regard to this. Some of the depressed people I've known have often convinced themselves that there's nothing fun to do anymore in life. It becomes 100% about work and that's it. So, is it any wonder that these people have depression issues?

To get out of this mindset, here's a thought experiment: ask yourself *why* do we work? The answer for most people is freedom—everybody wants to be more free, but this is accomplished through earning more money. And so we're told if we toil away for another few years that sense of freedom we want will finally happen. Or, we're banking completely on when we get to retire, which means no fun until we're senior citizens!

So the real currency in life are happy moments together (whether with friends or family), freedom—and parties! This is why we're working, right? Well, I think people forget about this frequently, and they begin working just to be able to say they're working, instead of ever cashing in the reward that we're supposed to be reaping from everything we're doing.

So my final lesson about this is to party more. In fact, don't just party more, make it a part of your life.

The Road to Self-Acceptance

The road to self-acceptance can be a long and hard one. It involves many of the factors I've listed so far in this chapter, including getting in touch with your inner-child, as well as learning to live within the moment. You are taken off course when you begin to compare yourself to society's expectations, magazine cover standards for beauty, or ideas about how you "should" live your life versus what you know you'd rather be doing.

For some of us, self-acceptance takes a lot longer because there is an inner-pain that doesn't go away. Sometimes, this is created in childhood through feelings of inadequacy. Too many loved ones I've seen from abusive homes seem to carry this pain with them 24 hours a day, 7 days a week, hiding in their subconscious and influencing their behavior.

If this is your situation, two things I suggest are psychotherapy and hypnotherapy. A psychotherapist will provide you the tools for your logical, conscious mind to begin fixing these problems, while a hypnotherapist will try to directly influence your subconscious. This is important, because it's in the subconscious where these negative beliefs take stranglehold, hiding in our mental basements, where they affect the thoughts we generate without us even being aware of what's happening.

You'll know self-acceptance once you feel it, because it's a remarkable sensation. You no longer have to worry about minute details of how you are behaving, looking or thinking, and it becomes much easier to enter the flow state (see my first point "Finding the Moment").

Spirituality

It's amazing the research that's been done to directly link spirituality with a reduction in depression. A study published in *JAMA Psychiatry* showed that among 103 participants, those who placed greater emphasis on spirituality or religion were not only less depressed, but their brains matched their mindset through thicker cortexes that is apparently a physiological trait that develops among people with less depression[18].

But what is spirituality? I think it's simply how you view the world. The opposite of spirituality is to see the world in a completely mechanical way. In other words, we are all wind-up toys, consciousness is an accident, and our lives are cosmic jokes. This attitude also leads to "non spiritual" actions like putting priority on squashing people below you, accumulating as much money as possible before death, and generally being very materialistic in thought and nature. This is something most religions warn about in some way or another, including Buddhism and also philosophical practices like Taoism.

Spirituality in contrast could then mean seeing our lives as sacred, the universe as being mysterious and that we are aspects of the universe itself, and our own lives have special significance. To see your life as cosmically important means that adversity can be almost always interpreted as something that's part of some grand scheme. Your position in society and what peers think of you are immediately deemphasized. This is compared to a non-spiritually minded person, who in place of greater significance of meaning, may be drawing his or her entire sense of purpose from social and cultural expectations. I see this among people who desire above all else to become famous and get attention. To what end? It's purely the feeding of social expectations, and it's anti-Spiritual, as the end result bears no impact on a grand "divine" plan for your life or the lives of others.

---

[18] http://psychcentral.com/news/2014/01/19/how-spirituality-protects-the-brain-against-depression/64698.html

I don't know if spirituality in this sense can be directly taught. I think it involves personal transformation. The good news is that sometimes the catalyst for a transformation in this regard is depression. To connect the dots from the first chapter, consider the holistic benefits of depression itself. It is your physiology and your emotions telling you that something in your life is without harmony. The final piece of this puzzle could be what some call spirituality, which is simply your recognition of who and what you are—your essence, and your divine purpose in life.

Your depression could be a disconnection from who and what you really are, and what you are here to do. As you awaken to understand what this is, that compression that you feel on your psyche will alleviate, and from darkness you will suddenly find inspiration. It is not uncommon at all for depression to be the precursor to a major positive change in a person's life, and in that way perhaps one could even be thankful for such an ailment; recognizing that it, too, had served a purpose in the grand scheme of things.

Final Thoughts

We've reached the end of our journey. It is my hope that when all of these points are put together, from the philosophical, to the nutritious, to the holistic, there will be a profound effect on your depressive symptoms.

Depression in this age is something that is far too easy to slip into. For many of us, it's almost like walking a tightrope, with depression the outcome of just one misstep. Our very temporary lives must be enjoyed with a high level of aspiration, spiritual principles, compassion, and dedicated self-development so that our time is not devoured by a downward negative spiral.

A Message from Andrea

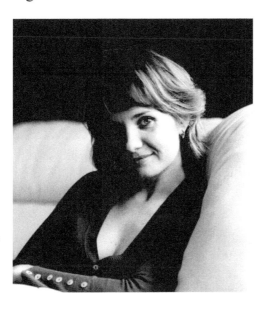

Thank you so much for taking the time to read this book. I hope that this was of some benefit to you.

You can find the rest of the books in this series by checking out www.developedlife.com/andreasilver. You can also reach me personally by e-mailing: AndreaSilverWellness@gmail.com.

A great book to with this one is my first in the series, *"30 Days to Amazing Health"*. In this book, I talk about the dangers of downward vortices for our emotions, and practical steps to pull yourself out of a psychological rut and obtain inner success.

Here is a preview:

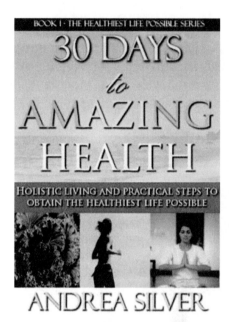

The Subconscious

Sometimes negative feelings also penetrate into our subconscious mind. And this is where the real danger lies, because while our subconscious regulates countless daily activities, we do not have direct control over it.

To best understand the subconscious, consider every thought you produce is sent into a type of *Cloud* hard-drive. If you imagine a teddy bear (you just did while reading this, because I queued it), consider that although the thought only appeared in your mind for a moment, it's *still there* in the Cloud drive, hidden from view. This is why sometimes we'll dream about strange obscure things we saw or thought about when we were awake, as this is when our mind begins exploring its hard drive, and all the strange junk sitting around inside of that attic.

Some ideas in the subconscious get stuck in there and could hurt our health from behind the scenes. As an example, you may have a strong subconscious belief that you are unhealthy, and despite outside evidence to the contrary, your "wiring" is still programmed to believe this. Childhood experiences often affect the subconscious the deepest, and if you were told (and believed) you were sickly or unhealthy as a child, it's likely that this state of mind has continued. And, from what we now understand about the mind's power—it could even be keeping you sick.

There are a few ways to address the subconscious:

Hypnosis: The practice of hypnosis is designed around directly influencing the subconscious mind. This is why hypnotherapy is often prescribed for patients with troubled childhoods and toxic subconscious beliefs that seem to linger behind the scenes. A hypnotherapist understands how to talk directly to a person's subconscious in a way that fixes problems.

Visualizing Before Sleep: When we sleep, our subconscious mind comes to the surface, and our waking mind is pushed aside, which is why we may experience images or even storylines, but we seemingly do not have the ability to control them or maintain regular consciousness (except in the case of lucid dreaming). So one trick I've learned through some meditation gurus I trained under is to practice your visualizations just as you're drifting to sleep; preferably right in that "in-between" state. Some people even do their visualizations *while* asleep by practicing lucid dreaming.

Evidence Gathering: Our subconscious likes to "gather evidence" about things to reinforce a belief. For an example, if you are socially shy and you walk into a crowded room, you may believe people are judging you. Then, when someone gives you a funny look (for whatever random reason), you will immediately interpret that as evidence to reinforce what you're telling yourself, and then you will become even worse off. Try to take control of these subconscious processes by looking for signs and evidence to create a positive narrative that you've created for yourself. It could be "I am healthy and attractive", and when someone looks at you—consider instead that they're admiring you!~

Discover how you can totally turn your life around in just 30 days by ordering your copy of "30 Days to Amazing Health" at www.developedlife.com/andreasilver

Free Gift: Also at the Andrea Silver page on Developed Life, don't forget to sign-up for my free PDF e-book companion, *The 20 Most Deceptive Health Foods*, which will educate you on the dishonest health food brands and the truly healthy alternatives.

Until next time,

More By Developed Life Books

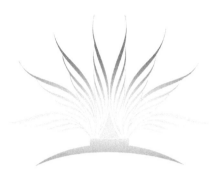

You can find more books at the following address: www.developedlife.com/bookstore.

Until next time!

Printed in France by Amazon
Brétigny-sur-Orge, FR

22973673R00040